Daily
Asthma
Logbook

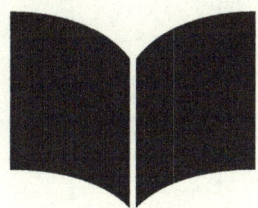

This book belongs to:

_____

Daily Logbook

Year	
Month	

Notes
_____
_____

Date/Time	Symptoms	Triggers	Weather	Treatment/Medication
				_____ _____
				_____ _____
				_____ _____
				_____ _____
				_____ _____
				_____ _____
				_____ _____

Daily Logbook

Year	
Month	

Notes
_____
_____

Date/Time	Symptoms	Triggers	Weather	Treatment/Medication
				_____ _____
				_____ _____
				_____ _____
				_____ _____
				_____ _____
				_____ _____
				_____ _____

Daily Logbook

Year	
Month	

Date/Time	Symptoms	Triggers	Weather	Treatment/Medication

Daily Logbook

Year	
Month	

Date/Time	Symptoms	Triggers	Weather	Treatment/Medication
				_____ _____
				_____ _____
				_____ _____
				_____ _____
				_____ _____
				_____ _____
				_____ _____

Daily Logbook

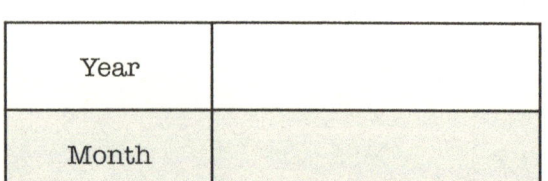

Year		
Month		

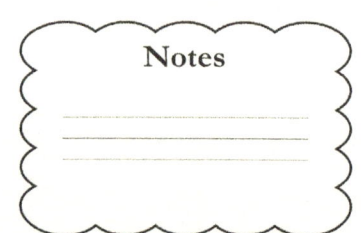

Notes

Date/Time	Symptoms	Triggers	Weather	Treatment/Medication

Daily Logbook

Year	
Month	

Notes
_____
_____
_____

Date/Time	Symptoms	Triggers	Weather	Treatment/Medication
				_____ _____
				_____ _____
				_____ _____
				_____ _____
				_____ _____
				_____ _____
				_____ _____

Daily Logbook

Year	
Month	

Notes

_____
_____

Date/Time	Symptoms	Triggers	Weather	Treatment/Medication
				_____ _____
				_____ _____
				_____ _____
				_____ _____
				_____ _____
				_____ _____
				_____ _____

Daily Logbook

Year		
Month		

Notes
_____
_____

Date/Time	Symptoms	Triggers	Weather	Treatment/Medication
				_____ _____
				_____ _____
				_____ _____
				_____ _____
				_____ _____
				_____ _____
				_____ _____

Daily Logbook

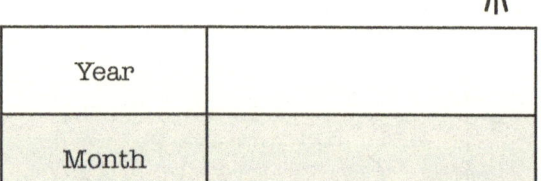

Year	
Month	

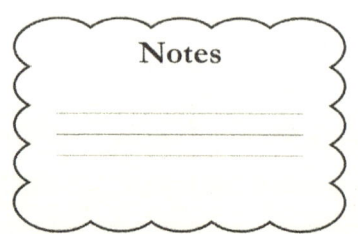

Notes

Date/Time	Symptoms	Triggers	Weather	Treatment/Medication

Daily Logbook

Year	
Month	

Notes

_____
_____
_____

Date/Time	Symptoms	Triggers	Weather	Treatment/Medication
				_____ _____
				_____ _____
				_____ _____
				_____ _____
				_____ _____
				_____ _____
				_____ _____

Daily Logbook

Year	
Month	

Date/Time	Symptoms	Triggers	Weather	Treatment/Medication
				_____ _____
				_____ _____
				_____ _____
				_____ _____
				_____ _____
				_____ _____
				_____ _____

Daily Logbook

Year	
Month	

Notes
_____
_____
_____

Date/Time	Symptoms	Triggers	Weather	Treatment/Medication
				_____ _____
				_____ _____
				_____ _____
				_____ _____
				_____ _____
				_____ _____
				_____ _____

Daily Logbook

Year	
Month	

Notes

Date/Time	Symptoms	Triggers	Weather	Treatment/Medication

Daily Logbook

Year	
Month	

Date/Time	Symptoms	Triggers	Weather	Treatment/Medication

Daily Logbook

	Year	
	Month	

Date/Time	Symptoms	Triggers	Weather	Treatment/Medication
				_____ _____
				_____ _____
				_____ _____
				_____ _____
				_____ _____
				_____ _____
				_____ _____

Daily Logbook

Year	
Month	

Notes

Date/Time	Symptoms	Triggers	Weather	Treatment/Medication

Daily Logbook

Year	
Month	

Date/Time	Symptoms	Triggers	Weather	Treatment/Medication

Daily Logbook

Year	
Month	

Notes
_____
_____

Date/Time	Symptoms	Triggers	Weather	Treatment/Medication
				_____ _____
				_____ _____
				_____ _____
				_____ _____
				_____ _____
				_____ _____
				_____ _____

Daily Logbook

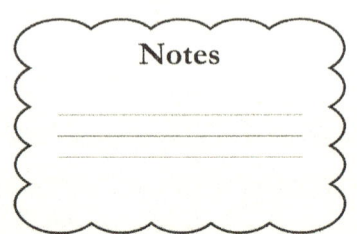

Year	
Month	

Date/Time	Symptoms	Triggers	Weather	Treatment/Medication

Daily Logbook

Year	
Month	

Notes

_____
_____

Date/Time	Symptoms	Triggers	Weather	Treatment/Medication
				_____ _____
				_____ _____
				_____ _____
				_____ _____
				_____ _____
				_____ _____
				_____ _____

Daily Logbook

Year	
Month	

Date/Time	Symptoms	Triggers	Weather	Treatment/Medication

Daily Logbook

	Year	
	Month	

Notes
_____
_____
_____

Date/Time	Symptoms	Triggers	Weather	Treatment/Medication
				_____ _____
				_____ _____
				_____ _____
				_____ _____
				_____ _____
				_____ _____
				_____ _____

Daily Logbook

	Year	
	Month	

Notes
_____
_____

Date/Time	Symptoms	Triggers	Weather	Treatment/Medication
				_____ _____
				_____ _____
				_____ _____
				_____ _____
				_____ _____
				_____ _____
				_____ _____

Daily Logbook

Year	
Month	

Notes
_____
_____
_____

Date/Time	Symptoms	Triggers	Weather	Treatment/Medication
				_____ _____
				_____ _____
				_____ _____
				_____ _____
				_____ _____
				_____ _____ _____
				_____ _____

Daily Logbook

Notes

Year	
Month	

Date/Time	Symptoms	Triggers	Weather	Treatment/Medication

Daily Logbook

Year	
Month	

Notes

Date/Time	Symptoms	Triggers	Weather	Treatment/Medication

Daily Logbook

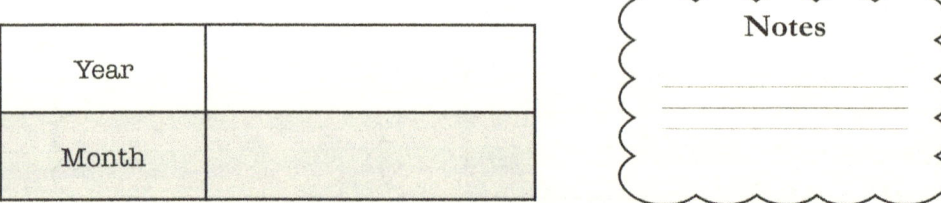

Year	
Month	

Notes
_____
_____

Date/Time	Symptoms	Triggers	Weather	Treatment/Medication

Daily Logbook

Year	
Month	

Date/Time	Symptoms	Triggers	Weather	Treatment/Medication
				_____ _____
				_____ _____
				_____ _____
				_____ _____
				_____ _____
				_____ _____
				_____ _____

Daily Logbook

Year	
Month	

Date/Time	Symptoms	Triggers	Weather	Treatment/Medication

Daily Logbook

Year	
Month	

Notes
_____
_____
_____

Date/Time	Symptoms	Triggers	Weather	Treatment/Medication
				_____ _____
				_____ _____
				_____ _____
				_____ _____
				_____ _____
				_____ _____
				_____ _____

Daily Logbook

Year	
Month	

Date/Time	Symptoms	Triggers	Weather	Treatment/Medication
				_____ _____
				_____ _____
				_____ _____
				_____ _____
				_____ _____
				_____ _____
				_____ _____

Daily Logbook

Year	
Month	

Notes

Date/Time	Symptoms	Triggers	Weather	Treatment/Medication

Daily Logbook

Year	
Month	

Notes

_____

_____

_____

Date/Time	Symptoms	Triggers	Weather	Treatment/Medication
				_____ _____
				_____
				_____
				_____ _____
				_____ _____
				_____ _____
				_____ _____

Daily Logbook

			Notes
Year			
Month			

Date/Time	Symptoms	Triggers	Weather	Treatment/Medication

Daily Logbook

Year	
Month	

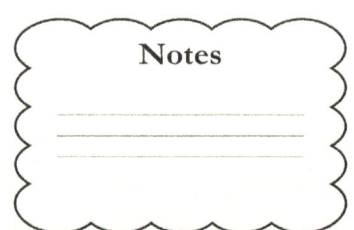

Date/Time	Symptoms	Triggers	Weather	Treatment/Medication

Daily Logbook

Year	
Month	

Notes
_____
_____

Date/Time	Symptoms	Triggers	Weather	Treatment/Medication
				_____ _____
				_____ _____
				_____ _____
				_____ _____
				_____ _____
				_____ _____
				_____ _____

Daily Logbook

Year	
Month	

Notes

_____
_____
_____

Date/Time	Symptoms	Triggers	Weather	Treatment/Medication
				_____ _____
				_____ _____
				_____ _____
				_____ _____
				_____ _____
				_____ _____
				_____ _____

Daily Logbook

Year	
Month	

Notes
_____
_____
_____

Date/Time	Symptoms	Triggers	Weather	Treatment/Medication
				_____ _____
				_____ _____
				_____ _____
				_____ _____
				_____ _____
				_____ _____
				_____ _____

Daily Logbook

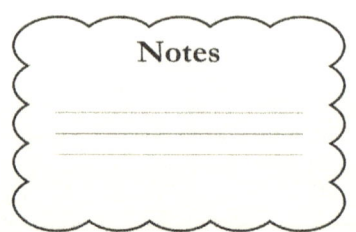

	Year	
	Month	

Date/Time	Symptoms	Triggers	Weather	Treatment/Medication

Daily Logbook

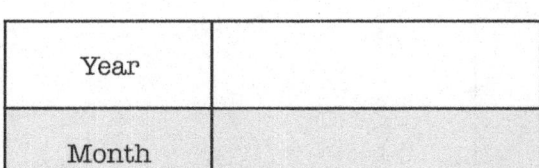

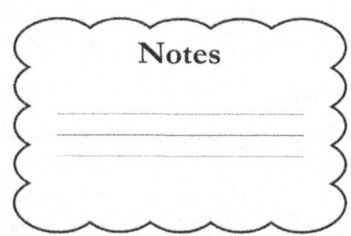

Year	
Month	

Notes

Date/Time	Symptoms	Triggers	Weather	Treatment/Medication

Daily Logbook

		Notes
Year		
Month		

Date/Time	Symptoms	Triggers	Weather	Treatment/Medication

Daily Logbook

Year	
Month	

Notes
_____
_____

Date/Time	Symptoms	Triggers	Weather	Treatment/Medication
				_____ _____
				_____ _____
				_____ _____
				_____ _____
				_____ _____
				_____ _____
				_____ _____

Daily Logbook

Year	
Month	

Notes

_____
_____
_____

Date/Time	Symptoms	Triggers	Weather	Treatment/Medication
				_____ _____
				_____ _____
				_____ _____
				_____ _____
				_____ _____
				_____ _____
				_____ _____

Daily Logbook

Year	
Month	

Notes
_____
_____
_____

Date/Time	Symptoms	Triggers	Weather	Treatment/Medication
				_____ _____
				_____ _____
				_____ _____
				_____ _____
				_____ _____
				_____ _____
				_____ _____

Daily Logbook

Year	
Month	

Date/Time	Symptoms	Triggers	Weather	Treatment/Medication

Daily Logbook

Year	
Month	

Notes

_____
_____
_____

Date/Time	Symptoms	Triggers	Weather	Treatment/Medication
				_____ _____
				_____ _____
				_____ _____
				_____ _____
				_____ _____
				_____ _____
				_____ _____

Daily Logbook

Year	
Month	

Date/Time	Symptoms	Triggers	Weather	Treatment/Medication

Daily Logbook

	Year	
	Month	

Notes
_____
_____
_____

Date/Time	Symptoms	Triggers	Weather	Treatment/Medication
				_____ _____
				_____ _____
				_____ _____
				_____ _____
				_____ _____
				_____ _____
				_____ _____

Daily Logbook

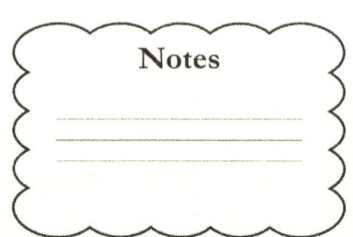

Year	
Month	

Date/Time	Symptoms	Triggers	Weather	Treatment/Medication

Daily Logbook

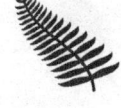

Year	
Month	

Notes

Date/Time	Symptoms	Triggers	Weather	Treatment/Medication

Daily Logbook

	Year	
	Month	

Date/Time	Symptoms	Triggers	Weather	Treatment/Medication
				_____ _____
				_____ _____
				_____ _____
				_____ _____
				_____ _____
				_____ _____
				_____ _____

Daily Logbook

Year	
Month	

Notes

Date/Time	Symptoms	Triggers	Weather	Treatment/Medication

Daily Logbook

	Year	
	Month	

Date/Time	Symptoms	Triggers	Weather	Treatment/Medication

Daily Logbook

Year	
Month	

Notes

Date/Time	Symptoms	Triggers	Weather	Treatment/Medication

Daily Logbook

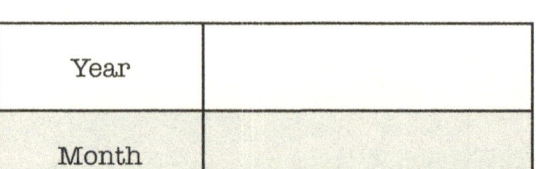

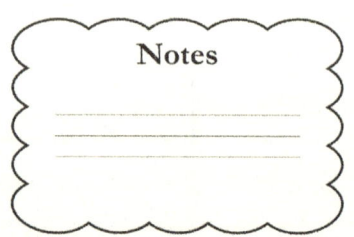

Year	
Month	

Notes

Date/Time	Symptoms	Triggers	Weather	Treatment/Medication

Daily Logbook

Year	
Month	

Notes

_____
_____

Date/Time	Symptoms	Triggers	Weather	Treatment/Medication
				_____ _____
				_____ _____
				_____ _____
				_____ _____
				_____ _____
				_____ _____
				_____ _____

Daily Logbook

Year	
Month	

Date/Time	Symptoms	Triggers	Weather	Treatment/Medication

Daily Logbook

	Year	
	Month	

Notes
_____
_____
_____

Date/Time	Symptoms	Triggers	Weather	Treatment/Medication
				_____ _____ _____
				_____ _____ _____
				_____ _____ _____
				_____ _____ _____
				_____ _____ _____
				_____ _____ _____
				_____ _____ _____

Daily Logbook

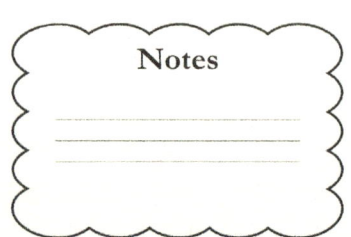

	Year	
	Month	

Date/Time	Symptoms	Triggers	Weather	Treatment/Medication
				_____ _____
				_____ _____
				_____ _____
				_____ _____
				_____ _____
				_____ _____
				_____ _____

Daily Logbook

Year	
Month	

Notes

Date/Time	Symptoms	Triggers	Weather	Treatment/Medication

Daily Logbook

Year	
Month	

Notes

Date/Time	Symptoms	Triggers	Weather	Treatment/Medication

Daily Logbook

Year	
Month	

Date/Time	Symptoms	Triggers	Weather	Treatment/Medication

Daily Logbook

Year	
Month	

Notes

_____
_____

Date/Time	Symptoms	Triggers	Weather	Treatment/Medication
				_____ _____
				_____ _____
				_____ _____
				_____ _____
				_____ _____
				_____ _____
				_____ _____

Daily Logbook

Year	
Month	

Date/Time	Symptoms	Triggers	Weather	Treatment/Medication
				_____ _____
				_____ _____
				_____ _____
				_____ _____
				_____ _____
				_____ _____
				_____ _____

Daily Logbook

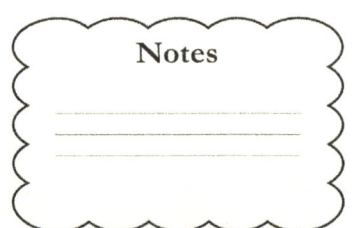

Year	
Month	

Notes

_____

_____

Date/Time	Symptoms	Triggers	Weather	Treatment/Medication
				_____ _____
				_____ _____
				_____ _____
				_____ _____
				_____ _____
				_____ _____
				_____ _____

Daily Logbook

Year	
Month	

Notes

Date/Time	Symptoms	Triggers	Weather	Treatment/Medication

Daily Logbook

Year	
Month	

Notes
_____
_____
_____

Date/Time	Symptoms	Triggers	Weather	Treatment/Medication
				_____ _____
				_____ _____
				_____ _____
				_____ _____
				_____ _____
				_____ _____
				_____ _____

Daily Logbook

Year	
Month	

Notes

_____
_____
_____

Date/Time	Symptoms	Triggers	Weather	Treatment/Medication
				_____ _____
				_____ _____
				_____ _____
				_____ _____
				_____ _____
				_____ _____
				_____ _____

Daily Logbook

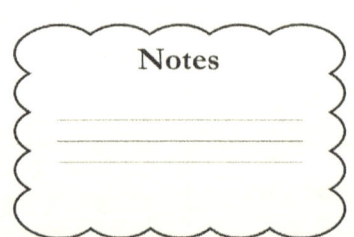

	Year	
	Month	

Notes
_____
_____

Date/Time	Symptoms	Triggers	Weather	Treatment/Medication
				_____ _____
				_____ _____
				_____ _____
				_____ _____
				_____ _____
				_____ _____
				_____ _____

Daily Logbook

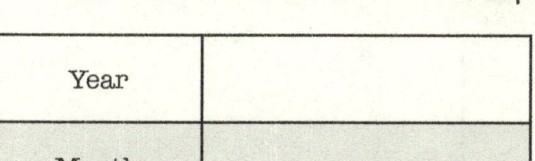

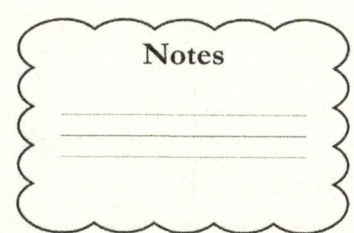

	Year	
	Month	

Notes
_____
_____
_____

Date/Time	Symptoms	Triggers	Weather	Treatment/Medication

Daily Logbook

Year	
Month	

Date/Time	Symptoms	Triggers	Weather	Treatment/Medication

Daily Logbook

Year	
Month	

Notes
_____
_____
_____

Date/Time	Symptoms	Triggers	Weather	Treatment/Medication
				_____ _____
				_____ _____
				_____ _____
				_____ _____
				_____ _____
				_____ _____
				_____ _____

Daily Logbook

Year	
Month	

Notes

Date/Time	Symptoms	Triggers	Weather	Treatment/Medication

Daily Logbook

Year	
Month	

Date/Time	Symptoms	Triggers	Weather	Treatment/Medication

Daily Logbook

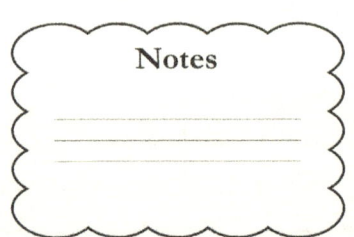

	Year	
	Month	

Date/Time	Symptoms	Triggers	Weather	Treatment/Medication

Daily Logbook

Year	
Month	

Date/Time	Symptoms	Triggers	Weather	Treatment/Medication

Daily Logbook

	Year	
	Month	

Notes
_____
_____

Date/Time	Symptoms	Triggers	Weather	Treatment/Medication
				_____ _____
				_____ _____
				_____ _____
				_____ _____
				_____ _____
				_____ _____
				_____ _____

Daily Logbook

Year	
Month	

Notes

Date/Time	Symptoms	Triggers	Weather	Treatment/Medication

Daily Logbook

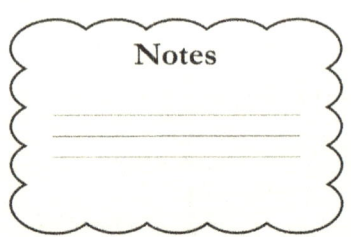

Year	
Month	

Date/Time	Symptoms	Triggers	Weather	Treatment/Medication
				_____ _____
				_____ _____
				_____ _____
				_____ _____
				_____ _____
				_____ _____
				_____ _____

Daily Logbook

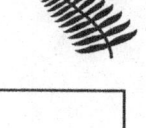

Year	
Month	

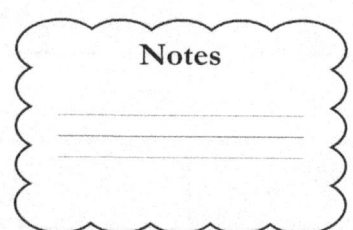

Notes

Date/Time	Symptoms	Triggers	Weather	Treatment/Medication

Daily Logbook

Year	
Month	

Notes

_____
_____

Date/Time	Symptoms	Triggers	Weather	Treatment/Medication
				_____ _____
				_____ _____
				_____ _____
				_____ _____
				_____ _____
				_____ _____
				_____ _____

Daily Logbook

		Notes
Year		
Month		

Date/Time	Symptoms	Triggers	Weather	Treatment/Medication

Daily Logbook

Year	
Month	

Notes
_____
_____
_____

Date/Time	Symptoms	Triggers	Weather	Treatment/Medication
				_____ _____
				_____ _____
				_____ _____
				_____ _____
				_____ _____
				_____ _____
				_____ _____

Daily Logbook

Year	
Month	

Notes

Date/Time	Symptoms	Triggers	Weather	Treatment/Medication

Daily Logbook

Year	
Month	

Notes

Date/Time	Symptoms	Triggers	Weather	Treatment/Medication

Daily Logbook

Year	
Month	

Notes

Date/Time	Symptoms	Triggers	Weather	Treatment/Medication

Daily Logbook

	Year	
	Month	

Notes
_____
_____

Date/Time	Symptoms	Triggers	Weather	Treatment/Medication
				_____ _____ _____
				_____ _____
				_____
				_____ _____
				_____ _____
				_____ _____
				_____ _____

Daily Logbook

Year	
Month	

Notes
_____
_____

Date/Time	Symptoms	Triggers	Weather	Treatment/Medication
				_____ _____
				_____ _____
				_____ _____
				_____ _____
				_____ _____
				_____ _____
				_____ _____

Daily Logbook

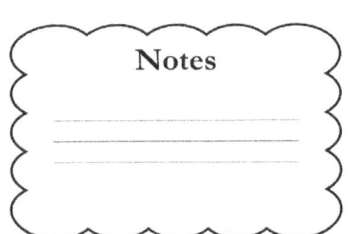

Year	
Month	

Notes

Date/Time	Symptoms	Triggers	Weather	Treatment/Medication

Daily Logbook

Year	
Month	

Notes

Date/Time	Symptoms	Triggers	Weather	Treatment/Medication

Daily Logbook

Year	
Month	

Date/Time	Symptoms	Triggers	Weather	Treatment/Medication
				_____ _____
				_____ _____
				_____ _____
				_____ _____
				_____ _____
				_____ _____
				_____ _____

Daily Logbook

Year		
Month		

Notes

_____
_____

Date/Time	Symptoms	Triggers	Weather	Treatment/Medication
				_____ _____
				_____ _____
				_____ _____
				_____ _____
				_____ _____
				_____ _____
				_____ _____

Daily Logbook

	Year	
	Month	

Notes

Date/Time	Symptoms	Triggers	Weather	Treatment/Medication

Daily Logbook

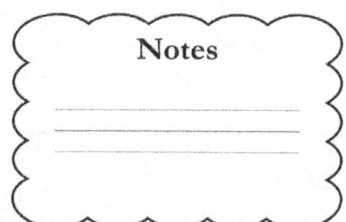

	Year	
	Month	

Notes

_____

_____

Date/Time	Symptoms	Triggers	Weather	Treatment/Medication
				_____ _____
				_____ _____
				_____ _____
				_____ _____
				_____ _____
				_____ _____
				_____ _____

Daily Logbook

Year	
Month	

Notes
_____
_____
_____

Date/Time	Symptoms	Triggers	Weather	Treatment/Medication
				_____ _____
				_____ _____
				_____ _____
				_____ _____
				_____ _____
				_____ _____
				_____ _____

Daily Logbook

Year	
Month	

Date/Time	Symptoms	Triggers	Weather	Treatment/Medication

Daily Logbook

Year	
Month	

Date/Time	Symptoms	Triggers	Weather	Treatment/Medication

Daily Logbook

Year	
Month	

Notes

Date/Time	Symptoms	Triggers	Weather	Treatment/Medication

Daily Logbook

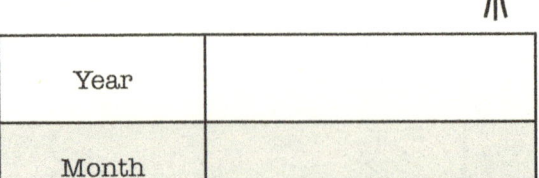

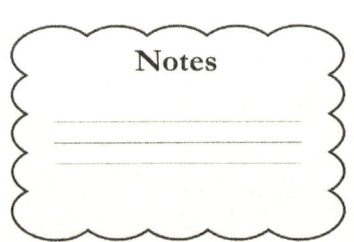

Year	
Month	

Notes

Date/Time	Symptoms	Triggers	Weather	Treatment/Medication

Daily Logbook

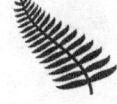

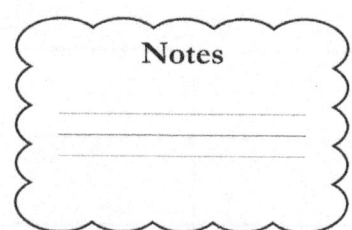

Year	
Month	

Notes
_____
_____
_____

Date/Time	Symptoms	Triggers	Weather	Treatment/Medication
				_____ _____
				_____ _____
				_____ _____
				_____ _____
				_____ _____
				_____ _____
				_____ _____

Daily Logbook

Year	
Month	

Notes

Date/Time	Symptoms	Triggers	Weather	Treatment/Medication

Daily Logbook

Year	
Month	

Notes
_____
_____
_____

Date/Time	Symptoms	Triggers	Weather	Treatment/Medication
				_____ _____
				_____ _____
				_____ _____
				_____ _____
				_____ _____
				_____ _____
				_____ _____

Daily Logbook

Year	
Month	

Notes
_____
_____
_____

Date/Time	Symptoms	Triggers	Weather	Treatment/Medication
				_____
				_____
				_____
				_____
				_____
				_____
				_____
				_____
				_____
				_____
				_____
				_____
				_____
				_____

Daily Logbook

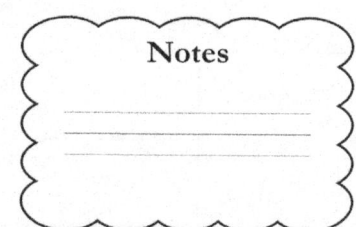

Year	
Month	

Date/Time	Symptoms	Triggers	Weather	Treatment/Medication

Daily Logbook

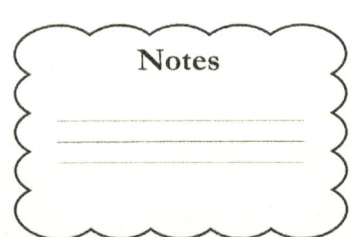

	Year	
	Month	

Notes
_____
_____
_____

Date/Time	Symptoms	Triggers	Weather	Treatment/Medication
				_____ _____
				_____ _____
				_____ _____
				_____ _____
				_____ _____
				_____ _____
				_____ _____

Daily Logbook

Year	
Month	

Notes

Date/Time	Symptoms	Triggers	Weather	Treatment/Medication

Daily Logbook

Year	
Month	

Date/Time	Symptoms	Triggers	Weather	Treatment/Medication

Daily Logbook

Year	
Month	

Notes

Date/Time	Symptoms	Triggers	Weather	Treatment/Medication

Daily Logbook

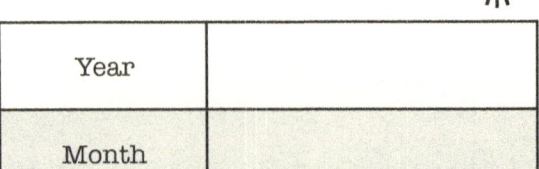

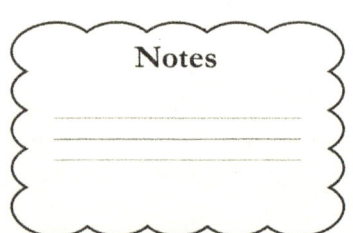

Year	
Month	

Notes
_____
_____
_____

Date/Time	Symptoms	Triggers	Weather	Treatment/Medication
				_____ _____
				_____ _____
				_____ _____
				_____ _____
				_____ _____
				_____ _____
				_____ _____

Daily Logbook

Year	
Month	

Notes

_____
_____
_____

Date/Time	Symptoms	Triggers	Weather	Treatment/Medication

Made in the USA
Coppell, TX
30 June 2021